CHAIR YOGA FOR SENIORS OVER 60 TO LOSE WEIGHT

Easy to follow Low impact Exercise to Enhance posture,Core Strength,Flexibility and balance 7 minutes Daily

Abel C. Kendricks

TABLE OF CONTENT

INTRODUCTION

In the middle of a busy metropolis lived a guy named Alejandro. He was once a dynamic guy constantly on the go, investigating the world around him with limitless enthusiasm.

However, as time went on, Alejandro became increasingly confined to his desk, preoccupied by the demands of his sedentary existence. Days passed into weeks, and weeks into months, until Alejandro recognized he was no longer the vibrant person he once was.

It started with minor hints, a twinge here and an ache there. Those clues quickly turned into constant discomforts, general body aching, tiredness that appeared to permeate into his bones, and joint pain that made even the most basic chores difficult. Stiffness crept into his joints, limiting his motions and lowering his spirits. Alejandro felt stuck in his own body, wishing to be free of the constraints of his sedentary existence.

On a fateful day, Alejandro stumbled upon this book, chair yoga for Seniors over 60 to lose weight, which would forever change the trajectory of his health.Intrigued by the promise of regeneration, Alejandro nervously glanced over its pages, dubious yet optimistic that there could be a ray of light despite his difficulties.

As Alejandro delved deeper into this book, he discovered a treasure mine of wisdom and instruction, painstakingly constructed to cater to people like himself, those afflicted by the wear and tear of time but yearning for renewal. Each page revealed a world of soft motions and focused breathing, designed expressly to relieve Alejandro's aches and pains.

With newfound motivation, Alejandro began practicing health, applying the hidden principles revealed inside the pages of this book. He enthusiastically embraced the practice of chair yoga, allowing its gentle embrace to re energize his tired muscles. Day by day, he felt the knots of anxiety unwind, replaced with a renewed sense of ease and vigor.

As the weeks grew into months, Alejandro marveled at the metamorphosis taking place within him. The once-stiff joints now moved fluidly, free of the limitations of immobility. The tiredness that had held him down was gone, replaced with an endless strength that powered his every movement. With each passing day, Alejandro felt himself regaining not just physical strength but also a zest for living.

Alejandro escaped from the shadows of his sedentary existence thanks to the power of chair yoga, demonstrating the human spirit's persistence and the transforming potential of conscious movement. And as he went on his trip, he carried renewed vigor and a deep appreciation for the simple yet profound gift of movement.

CHAPTER ONE

How Chair Yoga Can Help with Weight Loss

For starters, chair yoga encourages enhanced mobility and flexibility, which is very important for seniors. Seniors can enhance their range of motion by stretching and moving gently while seated, making it simpler to participate in other types of exercise.

Chair yoga strengthens muscles in the core, arms, and legs. As muscle mass rises, the body's metabolism improves, resulting in weight reduction. Stronger muscles promote better posture, which can reduce pain and make physical tasks simpler to complete.

Chair yoga also emphasizes deep breathing and relaxation methods, which can help relieve stress. High stress levels can cause weight gain by increasing cortisol production, which leads to cravings for unhealthy foods. Chair yoga, which incorporates mindfulness techniques, helps seniors manage stress and make better decisions.

Chair yoga can help improve circulation and digestion. Better circulation means that nutrients are distributed more efficiently throughout the body, whilst better digestion ensures that food is adequately absorbed and removed, decreasing bloating and assisting in weight control.

Consistency is essential in any weight reduction journey, and chair yoga provides a low-impact, accessible option that seniors can easily integrate into their daily routine. Whether it's a quick session in the morning or a few minutes before bed, consistent practice can provide big improvements over time.

Chair yoga for seniors over 60 can help them lose weight by improving mobility, building muscular strength, lowering stress, supporting improved circulation and digestion, and giving a practical exercise choice for regular practice. So, try including chair yoga into your daily practice to help you lose weight and improve your overall health.

Importance of Weight Loss for Seniors

Losing extra weight can improve older persons general health and quality of life. Excess weight puts strain on joints, worsens pre-existing health diseases such as diabetes and heart disease, and raises the risk of mobility problems and falls. Excess weight might result in diminished energy and independence.

Weight loss for seniors is about more than simply looking good; it's also about enhancing functioning and longevity. Seniors who embrace healthy living practices, such as frequent physical exercise and appropriate eating choices, can not only lose weight but also increase their strength, flexibility, and endurance.

This, in turn, can improve their capacity to carry out everyday tasks and lead an active, independent lifestyle.

Chair yoga is a great alternative for seniors who want to reduce weight safely and successfully. This mild type of yoga is suitable for people of all fitness levels and may be tailored to accommodate mobility constraints or health issues. Chair yoga emphasizes gentle stretching, breathing exercises, and mindfulness as a low-impact but effective technique to enhance flexibility, balance, and muscular tone.

Seniors who consistently participate in chair yoga sessions can burn calories, gain lean muscle mass, and enhance their general feeling of well-being. Chair yoga promotes relaxation and stress reduction, which can assist counteract emotional eating and improve long-term weight loss attempts.

Chair yoga may be included in a complete weight loss plan for seniors, providing considerable physical and emotional advantages. Chair yoga is an effective technique for promoting healthy aging and enhancing overall quality of life because it addresses the specific demands and obstacles that older individuals face.

Understanding the Benefits of Chair Yoga

Low-Impact workout: Chair yoga is a gentle, low-impact workout that is great for seniors who have mobility limitations or joint discomfort. It enables you to engage in physical activities without placing stress on your body. Chair yoga improves flexibility and range of motion. This is critical for elders since it can help avoid injuries and enhance daily mobility.

Muscle Strengthening: Even though chair yoga postures are seated, they activate multiple muscle groups, assisting in their long-term strength. Building muscle mass can help you lose weight by raising your metabolism and calorie burn, even while you're not moving.

Improves Balance and Stability: As we age, balance becomes increasingly vital for avoiding falls and injuries. Chair yoga combines postures and exercises to improve balance and stability, lowering the chance of injury.

Stress Reduction: Chair yoga incorporates breathing exercises and relaxation techniques to lower stress levels. Lower stress levels can result in better sleep and digestion, both of which can help with weight reduction.

Chair yoga promotes mindfulness and self-awareness: by strengthening the mind-body connection. This can lead to healthier lifestyle choices, such as food adjustments that aid weight loss efforts.

Supports Cardiovascular Health: While chair yoga may not be as rigorous as typical cardiovascular activities, it nevertheless delivers advantages for heart health. Gentle motions and regulated breathing can enhance circulation and reduce blood pressure, lowering your risk of heart disease.

Chair yoga may be practiced in almost any place, making it accessible and easy for elders. Chair yoga may be readily incorporated into your daily routine, whether at home, in a community center, or even at work, to help you lose weight.

It is a comprehensive approach to weight loss that improves physical fitness, mental well-being, and general quality of life. Regular practice can result in considerable increases in health and vigor.

Addressing Common Concerns and Misconceptions

"It's not intense enough": While Chair Yoga may appear to be less vigorous, it can still be useful for weight reduction. The regulated motions and poses activate muscles, improve flexibility, and increase general mobility, all of which help with calorie burn and weight management.

"It's only for relaxation": While Chair Yoga promotes relaxation and stress reduction, it is also an effective type of exercise. It includes dynamic movements, stretches, and strength-building positions, making it an ideal exercise program for seniors wanting to lose weight.

"I won't see results": Consistency is essential. Committing to regular Chair Yoga practices, combined with a healthy diet, can provide obvious improvements over time. Weight reduction may be slow, but the long-term advantages, such as improved posture, muscular tone, and energy levels, will increase overall well-being.

"It's too easy": Chair Yoga adapts classic yoga postures to seniors' requirements, making it both accessible and difficult. Variations and changes appeal to various fitness levels, resulting in an appropriate workout that aids weight reduction without strain or pain.

"I need cardio to lose weight": While cardio workouts are helpful, Chair Yoga is a low-impact option that supplements cardiovascular activities. Its emphasis on conscious movement, breath awareness, and gentle stretching encourages fat loss, muscular tone, and cardiovascular health.

"I'm too old to start": Your age should not prevent you from enjoying the advantages of Chair Yoga. Its mild approach reduces the chance of damage while promoting empowerment and self-care. It's never too late to put your health first and begin on a road to weight loss and vitality.

Chair Yoga for Seniors Over 60 is a comprehensive and successful weight reduction program that addresses common worries and misunderstandings by providing a gentle yet impacting workout regimen adapted to their specific goals and abilities.

When you approach the practice with an open mind and devotion, you will realize that it can improve both your body and your mind.

Setting Realistic Expectations

Setting realistic expectations is essential when beginning any fitness journey, particularly with chair yoga for seniors over 60 who want to reduce weight. First and foremost, keep in mind that weight loss is a gradual procedure with no guaranteed outcomes. It is critical to create realistic objectives based on your current fitness level, health status, and lifestyle.

Recognize that chair yoga has several benefits outside weight reduction, such as increased flexibility, balance, and mental well-being. Therefore, focus on total health improvement rather than just the number on the scale. Be patient and persistent in your approach, recognizing that little, incremental adjustments contribute to long-term success.

Understand your body's limitations and adjust your chair yoga practice accordingly. Listen to your body and don't push yourself too hard, especially if you're new to fitness or have any health difficulties. Consult a healthcare expert or a trained yoga instructor to create a safe and effective regimen that meets your specific needs.

Set clear, quantifiable, and realistic goals for your weight reduction journey. Instead of striving for quick weight reduction, strive for slow and sustainable progress, such as dropping 1-2 pounds each week. This strategy is healthier and more manageable in the long term.

Embrace the notion of non-scale successes, like higher energy levels, better posture, or fitting into lower clothes sizes. Celebrate your accomplishments along the road to keep motivated and inspired.

Keep focused on your chair yoga practice and lifestyle improvements. Consistency is essential for meeting and sustaining weight reduction goals.

Making realistic expectations, recognizing the advantages of chair yoga beyond weight loss, listening to your body, making manageable objectives, enjoying non-scale wins, and remaining dedicated can help you begin on a successful weight reduction path customized to your requirements as a senior over 60.

CHAPTER TWO

Getting Started with Chair Yoga

Starting with Chair Yoga for Seniors Over 60 to Lose Weight is a good decision since it provides a moderate yet effective approach to exercise. Here's a complete handbook to help you begin this adventure:

Choose the Right Chair: Select a solid, armless chair with a flat seat and backrest. This promotes stability and good posture during workouts.

Warm-up: Start with simple sitting motions to warm up your muscles and joints. Rotate your neck, shoulders, wrists, and ankles to improve circulation and flexibility.

Deep breathing exercises might help you oxygenate your body and relax your thoughts. Inhale deeply through your nose, filling your stomach, and exhale slowly through your mouth.

Basic Chair Yoga Poses: Begin with the sitting mountain posture, seated forward fold, and seated twist. These postures enhance posture, promote mobility, and strengthen the core muscles.

Progressive Movements: Gradually progress to more difficult postures as your strength and flexibility develop. Use positions like chair warrior, chair pigeon, and chair downward dog to work different muscle areas and improve weight reduction.

Mindful Awareness: Throughout your practice, be present and engaged, paying attention to your body's feelings and limits. Never push yourself too much, and always listen to your body.

Consistency is key. Encourage regular practice sessions, ideally three to five times per week. Consistency is key to seeing results and receiving the advantages of Chair Yoga for weight loss.

Chair Yoga should be used with a well-balanced diet that includes complete foods, lean meats, fruits, and vegetables. Hydration is also important, so consume lots of water throughout the day.

Seek Advice: If you're new to yoga or have any health issues, talk to a certified yoga instructor or a healthcare practitioner before beginning a new workout routine.

Enjoy the path: Embrace the path of self-discovery and growth. Celebrate your accomplishments, no matter how tiny, and be patient with yourself while working toward your weight reduction objectives.

Chair Yoga is a mild yet effective method of training for seniors over 60, promoting weight reduction, increasing flexibility, and improving general well-being. Enjoy your practice and gain from this fascinating kind of fitness.

Preparing Your Space and Equipment

To prepare your environment and equipment for chair yoga designed for seniors over 60 to help them lose weight, start by choosing a quiet, well-ventilated place with plenty of room to move. Remove any barriers or debris that may interfere with your exercise.

To avoid accidents, use a robust chair with no arms and place it on a non-slip surface. Place a yoga mat or non-slip towel beneath the chair for support and padding.

Next, collect your equipment. To integrate strength training into your program, use lightweight resistance bands or tiny hand weights. This will help with muscle toning and calorie burning. Also, have a water bottle handy to stay hydrated during your workout.

Dress appropriately by wearing comfortable, breathable clothes that allow for freedom of movement. Avoid clothing that is too loose or restricting, as this may interfere with your practice.

Before you start your chair yoga session, take a minute to set your objectives and goals. This mental preparation might help you maintain attention and motivation during the practice.

Throughout your practice, be aware of your body's limitations and alter postures as needed to meet any physical constraints or discomfort. Listen to your body and respect its demands, while avoiding pushing yourself too hard to avoid harm.

After completing your chair yoga practice, spend a few moments for gentle stretching and deep breathing to encourage relaxation and healing. Reflect on your practice and any success you've made toward your weight loss objectives.

Place your equipment in a dedicated location to keep your workspace neat and ready for future sessions. Regularly clean and examine your equipment to maintain its safety and lifespan. By deliberately organizing your environment and equipment, you can ensure a successful and pleasant chair yoga practice that promotes weight reduction and general well-being.

Choosing the Right Chair

When choosing a chair for Chair Yoga, consider comfort, support, and stability. Choose a chair with a straight back and solid construction to ensure appropriate alignment and prevent slouching during activity.

Look for chairs with cushioned seats and armrests to provide extra comfort during extended sessions. Ensure that the chair's height lets your feet rest flat on the ground, which will promote stability and balance during your practice.

Consider the chair's material as well. Choose a chair constructed of strong materials that can sustain repeated usage and give appropriate support for your body weight. Additionally, choose a chair with non-slip feet to avoid sliding or tipping during rapid motions.

For seniors over 60 trying to lose weight with Chair Yoga, look for a chair that meets their individual needs and limits. Look for chairs with larger seats and plenty of padding to comfortably accommodate people of all shapes and sizes. Prioritize seats with changeable characteristics, such as height and armrests, to tailor the chair to each individual's specific needs.

When considering possible seats, try them for comfort and stability. Sit in the chair for a lengthy amount of time to determine how comfortable it is and whether it gives appropriate support for your back and joints.

Pay attention to how the chair feels while performing various yoga poses and motions, maintaining optimal alignment and range of motion.

Selecting the appropriate chair for Chair Yoga is critical to optimize comfort, safety, and efficacy during practice. By picking a chair that suits your personal needs and preferences, you may have a satisfying and productive yoga session that is suited to your specific demands and objectives.

Clothing and Accessories for Comfort

When practicing Chair Yoga, especially for seniors over 60 who want to lose weight, choosing the correct attire and accessories is critical for comfort and safety. Choose breathable textiles like cotton or moisture-wicking materials to keep you comfortable and dry during your practice.

Loose-fitting clothing allows for unrestricted movement, increasing flexibility and mobility. Avoid wearing too tight clothes, which may limit circulation or produce pain.

Consider wearing layers that are easy to remove when your body temperature fluctuates during the session. This guarantees that you are comfortable and do not overheat or become too chilly. Wearing supportive undergarments can also help you feel more comfortable and confident during Chair Yoga sessions.

When it comes to accessories, consider investing in a high-quality yoga mat created exclusively for chair workouts. This offers cushioning and stability, lowering the chances of slipping or sliding during motions.

A yoga strap or resistance band can also help with stretching and flexibility, particularly for seniors who want to improve their range of motion and burn calories more effectively.

Consider wearing supportive footwear with non-slip soles for extra support and stability, particularly if you have mobility or balance challenges.

This helps to reduce slips and falls during Chair Yoga postures and transitions. However, if your practice consists mostly of sitting postures, bare feet or sticky socks may provide a greater connection with the chair and floor.

Always bring a water bottle to remain hydrated throughout your workout, since regular hydration is vital for peak performance and recovery. You may completely enjoy the advantages of Chair Yoga while still working towards your weight reduction goals if you wear the appropriate attire and accessories.

Warm-up and Stretching Exercises

Warm-up and stretching exercises are essential components of any workout regimen, especially for seniors over 60 who want to lose weight with Chair Yoga. Before starting the primary workout, you need to warm up your body properly.

Begin with mild motions that stimulate blood flow to your muscles and joints. This may involve marching in place, shoulder rolls, and mild arm swings. Next, focus on dynamic stretching exercises to relax your muscles and increase flexibility.

Leg swings, arm circles, and torso twists might help you prepare for your forthcoming workout. Dynamic stretching improves your range of motion and reduces injuries when exercising.

After your warm-up and dynamic stretching, go on to Chair Yoga positions designed specifically for seniors. These poses are moderate but beneficial for weight reduction and general fitness. Include motions like sat-forward bends, chair twists, and seated cat-cow stretches to stimulate your muscles and burn calories.

Throughout your Chair Yoga practice, try to breathe deeply and listen to your body. Modify positions to meet any physical limits or pain. Consistency is essential for losing weight and boosting fitness, so try to add Chair Yoga into your regimen at least a few times each week.

Warm-up and stretching activities are crucial for seniors over 60 who are participating in Chair Yoga for weight reduction. These preliminary motions boost blood flow, enhance flexibility, and lower the likelihood of damage during exercise. Incorporating dynamic stretching and Chair Yoga postures into your program allows you to reach your exercise objectives while emphasizing safety and enjoyment.

Breathing Techniques for Relaxation and Focus

To improve relaxation and attention via breathing methods, begin by choosing a comfortable sitting posture, such as in a chair for seniors over 60 doing Chair Yoga. Sit tall, keeping your spine straight but not stiff, allowing for natural curvature. Put your hands softly on your lap or thighs.

Begin by taking slow, deep breaths through your nose, allowing your abdomen to fully expand with each inhalation. Feel the breath flow into your lungs from the bottom up, expanding your chest and ribcage. As you exhale, let the air out slowly and thoroughly through your lips, feeling your abdomen gently constrict.

Concentrate on the sensation of the breath as it enters and departs your body, observing the rise and fall of your chest and belly with each inhale and exhale. Each exhale releases any tension or stress, enabling you to relax into the present now.

Incorporate mindfulness into your breathing practice by focusing on the present moment. Notice any ideas or feelings that occur without judgment, simply watching them as they come and go, gently returning your attention to the breath anytime you are distracted.

Experiment with several breathing methods to see what works best for you. Try alternate nostril breathing, which involves inhaling through one nostril while shutting the other with your thumb, then exhaling through the opposing nose, alternating sides with each breath.

Practice these breathing exercises regularly, including them in your daily routine to improve relaxation and attention. Over time, you'll discover that these approaches not only help you manage stress and anxiety but also boost your entire well-being and energy.

Tips for Incorporating Chair Yoga into Daily Routine

Incorporating chair yoga into your daily routine can help adults over 60 lose weight while increasing flexibility, strength, and general well-being. Here's a thorough guide on incorporating chair yoga into your daily life:

Begin slowly: Start with easy chair yoga postures to become used to the motions and prevent overexertion.

Set a Routine: Set aside set hours each day for your chair yoga practice to build consistency and habit.

Choose a peaceful Space: Locate a peaceful, clutter-free space where you may practice chair yoga without interruptions.

Invest in a Stable Chair: Make sure your chair is robust and stable enough to support your weight while you do various postures and exercises.

Warm Up: Start your chair yoga practice with simple stretches to get your muscles warmed up and ready for deeper poses.

Focus on Breathing: Throughout your practice, pay attention to your breath, breathing deeply with your nose and expelling completely through your mouth.

Explore Different Positions: Use a range of chair yoga positions to target different muscle groups and parts of the body.

Listen to your body. Respect your body's limitations and adjust postures as necessary to minimize strain or injury.

Gradually Increase Intensity: As you grow more comfortable with chair yoga, gradually increase the intensity and duration of your sessions to push yourself.

Stay Hydrated: Drink lots of water before, during, and after your chair yoga session to keep your body hydrated and aid in recovery.

Monitor your development by noticing increases in strength, flexibility, and overall well-being.

Stay Consistent: To receive the full advantages of chair yoga and meet your weight reduction objectives, stick to practice regularly.

By implementing these techniques into your daily practice, you may use chair yoga to improve your physical health and reach your weight reduction goals more efficiently.

CHAPTER THREE

Understanding the Basics of Chair Yoga

Understanding the fundamentals of Chair Yoga is critical, particularly for seniors over 60 wanting to reduce weight. Chair Yoga is a mild yet effective form of exercise that is suitable for anyone with restricted movement or balance concerns.

Begin by choosing a solid chair without arms and placing it on a non slip surface. Sit comfortably with your feet flat on the ground, keeping your spine and shoulders aligned. Begin with deep breathing techniques to ground yourself and prepare for movement.

Chair Yoga consists of a sequence of easy stretches and postures adjusted to be performed while seated or using the chair for support. These exercises target specific muscle areas, increasing flexibility, strength, and balance. Your mobility and range of motion will improve as you proceed.

Poses such as sitting forward bends, spinal twists and side stretches will stimulate core muscles and improve circulation. These motions also help digestion and release stress in the body.

Incorporate focused breathing into your practice to promote relaxation and minimize tension. Focusing on your breath enables you to deepen each stretch while remaining present in the moment.

Consistency is essential while practicing Chair Yoga for weight reduction. To see results, commit to at least 20-30 minutes of practice multiple times each week. As you grow more accustomed to the exercises, progressively increase the intensity and duration of your workouts.

Stay hydrated and listen to your body's cues. If you feel any discomfort or pain, alter your position or take a break. It's critical to accept your limitations and engage in self-care.

Chair Yoga provides seniors with a gentle yet effective technique to shed weight and enhance their overall health. Understanding the fundamentals and committing to a consistent practice will provide you with the advantages of enhanced strength, flexibility, and awareness.

What is Chair Yoga?

Chair yoga is a moderate type of yoga that involves performing conventional yoga postures while seated or supported by a chair. It is especially useful for seniors over 60 who may have mobility limitations or find it difficult to execute regular yoga positions on the mat.

Chair yoga is a sequence of mild stretches, twists, and breathing exercises that aim to enhance flexibility, strength, and balance. A chair offers stability and support, making it suitable for elders with restricted movement or balance issues.

This type of yoga encourages relaxation and stress reduction via regulated breathing and focused movement. It can help elders manage the symptoms of illnesses such as arthritis, osteoporosis, and chronic pain, as well as reduce stiffness and increase range of motion.

Chair yoga is a low-impact form of exercise that is appropriate for people who suffer from joint discomfort or other disabilities. Gentle motions and stretches can help to improve blood circulation, muscular tone, and general mobility.

For seniors over the age of 60 who want to reduce weight, chair yoga can be an important part of a comprehensive wellness plan. While chair yoga may not burn as many calories as high-intensity workouts, it can still help with weight reduction by encouraging mindfulness, lowering stress-related eating, and improving general physical activity.

Additionally, chair yoga helps enhance digestion and metabolism, both of which are important aspects of weight management. Seniors can lose weight gradually and enhance their general health and well-being by exercising regularly and adopting good eating habits.

Chair yoga provides seniors over 60 with a mild yet effective approach to keeping active, increasing flexibility, and supporting weight reduction objectives, all while reaping the many physical and mental health benefits of yoga.

History and Origins of Chair Yoga

Chair yoga is based on the ancient practice of yoga, which began in India over 5,000 years ago. Traditional yoga was mostly performed on the ground, but as the practice grew, modifications were made to suit people with physical limitations. Chair yoga was created to make yoga more accessible to people who may struggle with traditional postures due to age, injury, or mobility limitations.

The original origins of chair yoga are unknown, but it became popular in the West in the late twentieth century as part of a larger push to make yoga more inclusive and accessible to varied communities.

It was primarily designed as a type of rehabilitation treatment for those suffering from accidents or operations, as well as the elderly who want to preserve or enhance their mobility and general well-being.

Chair yoga is the practice of completing yoga postures and exercises while seated or supported on a chair. The practice includes moderate stretches, breathing methods, and mindfulness exercises, all of which can enhance flexibility, strength, balance, and mental clarity. In addition, chair yoga is a low-impact type of exercise that decreases the chance of strain or injury, making it suitable for seniors over 60.

Chair yoga may not be as strenuous as other types of exercise for weight reduction, but when paired with a balanced diet and lifestyle, it may be quite successful. Chair yoga can help with weight control by increasing calorie expenditure, improving metabolism, and promoting muscular tone.

Chair yoga is a modified version of conventional yoga that is both accessible and useful to seniors over the age of sixty. While not as strenuous as other types of exercise, chair yoga is a gentle and effective approach to enhance general health, and mobility, and may even aid in weight reduction when paired with other good habits.

Principles and Philosophy

First and foremost, the notion of flexibility must be understood. Fitness is not one-size-fits-all, especially for the elderly. Chair Yoga is a mild yet effective form of physical practice that may accommodate people with varied levels of mobility and flexibility.

Second, consistency is key. Encouraging elderly to practice Chair Yoga daily promotes moderate and long-term weight reduction. Consistency fosters habits that result in long-term success.

Thirdly, awareness is quite important. Chair Yoga focuses on the mind-body connection, encouraging awareness of sensations, breathing, and movement. Mindfulness not only improves exercise efficacy, but it also boosts general well-being.

Growth is vital. As seniors gain proficiency in Chair Yoga postures and routines, progressively increasing the intensity and duration of sessions promotes long-term improvement and weight loss.

Additionally, individualization is essential. Chair Yoga practices are tailored to each senior's specific requirements and skills, ensuring safety and maximizing outcomes. Personalized adaptations account for any physical limits or health concerns.

Community support increases motivation and satisfaction. Creating a friendly setting in which elders feel encouraged and respected increases adherence to Chair Yoga programs, making weight reduction more manageable and pleasurable.

Overall Well-being is addressed. While weight loss may be the primary aim, Chair Yoga for Seniors offers more than simply physical advantages. It promotes emotional, mental, and spiritual well-being, resulting in a balanced and fulfilled living.

Combining these ideas and philosophy into Chair Yoga for Seniors Over 60 to Lose Weight assures a comprehensive strategy that promotes adaptation, consistency, mindfulness, advancement, individualization, community support, and overall well-being.

Key Concepts and Terminology

When it comes to Chair Yoga for Seniors Over 60 Who Want to Lose Weight, several fundamental ideas and terminology are essential for comprehension and application.

Chair Yoga is a modified style of yoga in which postures and stretches are performed while seated on a chair or utilizing a chair as support. This modification makes it more accessible to people with mobility challenges or limits.

Weight loss is the process of losing body weight, which is often accomplished by a combination of food adjustments, exercise, and lifestyle alterations. Seniors should focus on long-term weight loss approaches that promote overall health and well-being.

Mobility refers to the capacity to move freely and effortlessly. Chair Yoga techniques are intended to increase mobility by gently stretching and strengthening muscles and joints, making them especially good for seniors who suffer from age-related stiffness or restrictions. The extent your muscles and joints can stretch to is called Flexibility

Chair Yoga improves flexibility through mild stretching movements, increasing mobility and lowering the chance of injury. Strength is the capacity of your muscles to apply force against the opposition. While Chair Yoga does not include traditional weight training, it does aid in developing muscle strength via various postures and motions that target different muscle areas.

Balance refers to the capacity to keep your body stable and under control. Chair Yoga incorporates exercises to enhance balance, which is essential for seniors to avoid falls and retain independence.

Mindfulness is the discipline of being present and aware of your thoughts, emotions, and experiences. Chair Yoga frequently involves mindfulness practices like deep breathing and meditation, which can help reduce stress and emotional eating, hence aiding with weight reduction attempts.

Adaptation is the process of modifying poses and exercises to meet the requirements and abilities of each individual. Adaptation is essential in Chair Yoga for Seniors to guarantee safety and efficacy while taking into consideration any physical limits or health issues.

Understanding these important principles and terminology will allow seniors to launch on their Chair Yoga journey with clarity and confidence, working toward their weight reduction objectives while emphasizing their entire health and well-being.

How Chair Yoga Differs from Traditional Yoga

Chair yoga varies from regular yoga in several important aspects, particularly for seniors over 60 looking to reduce weight. First, chair yoga is adapted to be practiced while seated or with the use of a chair, making it more accessible to people with restricted mobility or balance concerns. Traditional yoga sometimes requires standing or moving through various positions on a mat, which can be difficult for seniors with physical limitations.

Second, chair yoga focuses on moderate exercises and stretches that improve flexibility, strength, and balance, all of which are important for seniors' weight reduction. These motions are intended to be low-impact and safe, minimizing the risk of damage while delivering effective training.

Traditional yoga, on the other hand, may contain more aggressive sequences and postures that are too demanding or daunting for seniors, particularly those who are new to fitness or recuperating from ailments.

It combines breathing methods and mindfulness practices to encourage relaxation and stress reduction, which is essential for general health and weight control. Seniors frequently suffer elevated stress levels, which can lead to weight gain or difficulties in decreasing weight. Chair yoga, which incorporates relaxation methods, helps seniors handle stress more efficiently, therefore boosting their weight reduction journey.

Chair yoga programs are often tailored to the unique requirements and skills of seniors, with teachers providing adaptations and variations to fit individual variances. This tailored approach guarantees that seniors may safely participate and advance at their speed, without feeling overwhelmed or disheartened when compared to others in a regular yoga session.

Chair yoga is a gentle yet effective technique for seniors over 60 to improve their fitness, including weight reduction, by providing accessible, low-impact activities that promote safety, relaxation, and personalized instruction.

Benefits of Chair Yoga for Seniors

Chair yoga has various benefits for seniors over the age of 60 who want to reduce weight while also improving their general health and well-being. For starters, it offers a mild type of exercise that can be readily tailored to different mobility levels, making it accessible to seniors with restricted mobility or physical limitations.

Chair yoga improves flexibility, balance, and mobility, which are critical for retaining independence and lowering the risk of falling. Furthermore, the exercise reduces stiffness and joint discomfort that are typically linked with aging, allowing seniors to move more easily and participate in other physical activities.

Chair yoga encourages relaxation and stress reduction via deep breathing and mindfulness exercises. This is especially advantageous for seniors who may be stressed or anxious about their weight or other health issues. Chair yoga improves sleep quality and mental health by lowering stress levels.

Chair yoga can help you lose weight by improving your metabolism and burning more calories. While the practice is not as strenuous as traditional forms of exercise, frequent involvement can nonetheless help with progressive weight reduction and maintenance. Chair yoga also promotes attentive eating habits and increased awareness of hunger and fullness cues by cultivating a mind-body connection.

Chair yoga fosters a feeling of community and social connection since seniors may engage in group courses and interact with people who have similar aims and interests.

This social support helps keep seniors motivated and devoted to their health goals.

It provides a safe, convenient, and effective approach for seniors over 60 to increase their physical fitness, control their weight, and improve their overall quality of life. Seniors who include regular practice into their routine can reap a slew of advantages that will boost their health and well-being for years to come.

CHAPTER FOUR

Chair Yoga Poses for Weight Loss

Chair yoga postures are an excellent alternative for adults over 60 aiming to lose weight while increasing their general health and mobility. These postures provide mild yet effective motions that may be performed while seated in a chair, making them accessible to people of all fitness levels and flexibility.

Begin with sitting forward bends to stretch the hamstrings and lower back, which will increase flexibility and relieve stress. To warm up the spine and promote mobility, repeat chair cat-cow stretches.

Move into chair warrior postures to strengthen your legs, core, and arms while increasing your balance and stability.

Incorporate chair twists to promote digestion and cleansing, resulting in weight loss from the inside.

Don't forget about chair leg lifts, which focus on the core and leg muscles while increasing strength and endurance. Aim to hold each posture for 5-10 breaths, gradually increasing the time and intensity as you gain comfort. Consistency is essential, so include these chair yoga postures in your daily practice for at least 15-20 minutes every session.

Combine your chair yoga practice with a healthy diet high in whole foods, lean proteins, and lots of fruits and vegetables. In addition, regular cardiovascular activity might help you lose weight. Listen to your body and respect its limitations, pushing yourself just as far as you feel comfortable and safe.

Committing to a regular chair yoga practice, along with appropriate eating choices and physical activity, will help you lose weight while also improving your general well-being, energy levels, and quality of life. Accept the road and enjoy each tiny accomplishment along the way.

Seated Forward Fold (Paschimottanasana)

Seated Forward Fold, also known as Paschimottanasana, is a useful yoga position, especially for seniors over 60 who want to reduce weight with chair yoga. To do it, sit tall in a chair, feet hip-width apart and flat on the ground. Inhale deeply, stretching your spine.

As you exhale, bend forward from your hips, reaching your hands for your feet or the floor. Maintain a straight back and avoid curving your spine excessively.As you fold forward, stretch through the crest of your head and reach your chest toward your thighs.

Feel the stretch at the backs of your legs, especially the hamstrings and calves. Hold the position for a few breaths, using light pressure without causing discomfort.

Seated Forward Fold provides various advantages for seniors looking to lose weight. It stretches the spine, hamstrings, and calves, which improves flexibility and mobility. The posture also improves digestion and massages the abdominal organs, promoting a healthy metabolism.

Paschimottanasana relaxes the mind and decreases stress, which can help with weight reduction by reducing emotional eating and encouraging mindful eating practices. Regular practice of this position helps improve posture and ease tension in the back and neck, resulting in better overall health.

For seniors over the age of 60, chair yoga versions of Paschimottanasana offer accessibility and support while still providing considerable benefits. By including this posture in a chair yoga program, people may get the benefits of yoga practice without having to do difficult or rigorous motions, making it a great alternative for older adults looking to improve their fitness and manage their weight successfully.

Chair Warrior I (Virabhadrasana I)

Chair Warrior I, also known as Virabhadrasana I, is a strong yoga position that can help seniors over 60 lose weight using chair yoga. Start by sitting tall on a firm chair, feet level on the ground and hip-width apart. Keep your spine straight and your shoulders relaxed.

To begin Chair Warrior I, place your feet firmly on the floor. As you inhale, raise your arms upward, palms together or shoulder-width apart. To support your spine,engage your core muscles.

As you exhale, slowly twist your torso to the right, placing your right hand on the back of the chair and your left hand on your right thigh.

Deepen the twist by softly placing your left palm into your right thigh while maintaining spinal length. Lift your chest to the ceiling and look over your right shoulder while maintaining your neck aligned with your spine.

As you maintain the posture, concentrate on your breathing, taking deep inhales and exhales to promote oxygen flow to your muscles. Feel the stretch across your back, shoulders, chest, and hips. Hold the stance for 30 seconds to 1 minute before gently releasing and repeating on the opposing side.

Chair Warrior, improves flexibility, strength, and balance, making it an ideal workout for seniors who want to reduce weight. This position, which engages many muscle groups and promotes good alignment, can enhance calorie burn and metabolism. Furthermore, the gentle twisting action promotes digestion and helps to ease lower back pain.

Add Chair Warrior I to your chair yoga program 2-3 times per week, progressively increasing the duration and intensity as your strength and flexibility develop. Endeavor to listen to your body and adjust the position as needed for comfort and safety. As with any workout regimen, you should contact your doctor before beginning, especially if you have any pre-existing health concerns.

Chair Warrior II (Virabhadrasana II)

Chair Warrior II, also known as Virabhadrasana II, is a modified yoga posture that is ideal for seniors over 60 who want to lose weight and enhance their general fitness. Begin by sitting tall on a solid chair, your feet hip-width apart and firmly planted on the floor. Use your core muscles to stabilize your spine and keep appropriate posture throughout the position.

Begin by extending your right leg out to the side, with the foot flat on the ground. Your left leg stays bent at a 90-degree angle, with the knee immediately above the ankle. This stance resembles a broad leg stance as if a warrior were prepared for combat.

Next, stretch your arms out to the sides at shoulder height, parallel to the ground, palms facing down. Keep your shoulders relaxed and away from your ears, and focus your attention on your right fingertips, keeping your neck in line with your spine.

As you hold the posture, concentrate on deepening your breath and activating your legs, core, and arms. As you maintain the position, you will feel your body's strength and stability increase.

Chair Warrior II provides various benefits to elders, including increased balance, strength, and flexibility. It also helps to loosen the hips and stretch the inner thighs, groin, and chest muscles.

To deepen the position, bend your front knee slightly, keeping it aligned with the ankle. You may also try moving your eyes upward to challenge your balance and attention.

Repeat Chair Warrior II on both sides, maintaining the posture for several breaths on both to maintain balance and symmetry in your practice. As you adopt this position into your daily routine, you will experience greater energy, mobility, and weight reduction advantages.

Chair Twists for Digestion and Detoxification

Chair twists are an excellent approach to stimulate digestion and detoxification in your body, especially for seniors over 60 wanting to lose weight. When you practice chair twists, you engage your abdominal muscles and activate the internal organs, which aids digestion by increasing the flow of digestive fluids and alleviating bloating and pain.

To begin, sit tall in a solid chair, feet level on the ground, knees hip-width apart. Place your hands on the chair's armrests or sides for support. Inhale deeply, stretching your spine, and as you exhale, gently rotate your body to the right with your core muscles.

Place your left hand on the outside of your right leg and your right hand on the chair's backrest or behind you for support. Keep your shoulders relaxed and your chest open while holding the twist for a few breaths.

As you twist, you're not only wringing out toxins from your organs but also massaging and conditioning the abdominal region. This can assist improve bowel motions and relieve constipation, therefore promoting detoxification.

Always breathe deeply and evenly during the twist, which will help oxygen circulate freely to your organs and aid in the detox process. After a few moments, gently release the twist and return to the center. Twist the other side, this time to the left.

Including chair twists in your daily routine can improve your digestive health and general well-being. Along with a healthy diet and regular physical exercise, chair yoga positions like twists might help you lose weight, especially if you're over the age of 60.

Chair Squats for Lower Body Strength

To begin, Chair Squats are an excellent workout for increasing lower-body strength, particularly for seniors over 60 who want to lose weight. This exercise works essential muscular groups including the quadriceps, hamstrings, and glutes, improving overall stability and mobility.

To execute Chair Squats, sit on the edge of a solid chair, feet hip-width apart and firmly planted on the ground. Engage your core muscles and elevate your chest throughout the process.

Next, carefully get up from the chair, pushing through your heels and extending your hips and knees until you are standing. Keep your weight properly divided on both feet and avoid leaning too much forward or backward.

Once standing, stop briefly at the top of the action before carefully lowering yourself down to a sitting posture, maintaining control, and keeping your knees in line with your toes.

To avoid strain or injury, execute Chair Squats with perfect technique. Keep your back upright, chest raised, and knees in line with your toes throughout the exercise.

Chair Squats are a safe and efficient approach for adults over 60 to increase lower body strength without overworking their joints. Additionally, including Chair Yoga postures into your regimen helps improve flexibility and balance while also assisting in weight reduction.

Chair squats are an excellent complement to any exercise regimen, as they provide an easy and efficient technique for seniors to build lower body strength and support weight reduction objectives. When paired with Chair Yoga, these movements provide a comprehensive approach to well-being and vitality for people over 60.

Chair Sun Salutations for Cardiovascular Health

To begin, Chair Sun Salutations are an excellent way to improve cardiovascular health, especially for seniors over 60 looking to lose weight. This modified style of yoga offers a low-impact yet effective workout for people with restricted mobility or who prefer softer training regimens.

Chair Sun Salutations involve a repetitive flow of motions that raise your heart rate, improving cardiovascular endurance and circulation. Controlled breathing methods oxygenate your blood, improving overall heart health while also promoting relaxation and stress alleviation.

These chair-based workouts work several muscular areas, such as the arms, shoulders, core, and legs. Each action increases flexibility, strength, and balance, all of which are essential for preserving functional independence as you age. By combining dynamic stretches and postures, you may increase joint mobility and relieve stiffness, increasing overall mobility and lowering the risk of falling.

Chair Sun Salutations stimulate the lymphatic system, promoting cleansing and immunological function. As you progress through the sequences, you will increase blood flow to important organs, increasing digestion, metabolism, and toxin clearance, all of which contribute to weight control and general well-being.

Chair Sun Salutations are a safe and accessible way for seniors over 60 to boost their physical activity levels without putting themselves in danger of harm. Consistent practice can result in steady weight loss by burning calories, improving muscular tone, and increasing metabolism. Yoga also encourages attentive eating habits and increased awareness of hunger cues, which help long-term weight management objectives.

Chair Sun Salutations are a vital weapon in your exercise arsenal, providing a comprehensive approach to cardiovascular health and weight reduction that is adapted to the specific needs of seniors over the age of 60. Accept this practice as part of your wellness path and appreciate the myriad advantages it provides for the body, mind, and soul.

CHAPTER FIVE

Creating Effective Chair Yoga Routines

To design successful chair yoga routines for seniors over 60 who want to lose weight, focus on integrating moderate movements, stretches, and breathing exercises that build flexibility, strength, and awareness.

Begin each session with a modest warm-up to get the body ready for exercise and lower the chance of injury. Include sitting stretches that target key muscle groups including the shoulders, chest, hips, and legs to improve flexibility and range of motion.

Next, use strength-building workouts like resistance bands or small weights to boost muscular tone and metabolism. Include sitting postures such as seated forward bends, seated twists, and seated leg lifts to work the core and lower body muscles. To increase awareness and relaxation, focus on good alignment and breathing methods during each action.

To test balance and stability while developing the legs and core muscles, transition into standing postures with the chair as support if necessary. To increase lower body strength and endurance, incorporate exercises such as chair squats, chair lunges, and chair mountain poses.

Include fluid sequences that keep the body moving and the heart rate raised, such as sitting sun salutations or chair vinyasa flows. Encourage participants to move consciously and coordinate breath with movement to strengthen the mind-body connection and promote relaxation.

Finish each session with a relaxing cooldown that includes moderate stretches and relaxation methods to relieve tension and quiet the mind. Encourage participants to practice deep, diaphragmatic breathing to enhance relaxation and stress reduction.

Adjust the intensity and duration of each program to meet the particular demands and fitness levels of the participants. Offer adjustments and options to persons with mobility challenges or physical restrictions. Regular practice of these chair yoga practices, paired with a healthy diet, can help seniors over 60 lose weight, increase mobility, and enhance their general health.

Understanding the Components of a Routine

Understanding the components of a routine is critical for good fitness, especially when personalizing it to specific populations, such as seniors over 60 who practice chair yoga for weight reduction.

Warm-up: Start with easy motions to promote blood flow and prepare your muscles for action. Chair yoga warm-ups may involve neck rolls, shoulder shrugs, and moderate twists to release the spine.

Strength Exercises: Use resistance training to increase muscular growth and metabolism. Concentrate on activities that target main muscular groups, such as leg lifts, bicep curls with low weights, and sitting squats with the chair as support.

Cardiovascular Activity: Use low-impact cardio workouts to raise your heart rate and burn calories. Chair yoga exercises can incorporate dynamic movements such as sitting marching, arm circles, and modified jumping jacks to improve circulation and fat reduction.

.Stretching exercises can help you improve your range of motion and avoid injuries. Chair yoga positions such as sitting forward bends, moderate twists and side stretches promote flexibility and mobility, which aids weight loss attempts.

Balance Work: Focus on balance and stability to lessen the chance of falls and enhance general coordination. Incorporate chair yoga positions that require balance, such as tree pose or sitting eagle pose, to work core muscles and burn calories.

Cool down: Finish the workout with soothing activities to reduce your heart rate and encourage relaxation. Gentle stretches and deep breathing exercises can help seniors ease out of their workouts and decrease muscular stiffness.

Progression and Variation: Gradually increase the intensity and complexity of workouts to avoid plateaus and stay motivated. Introduce new motions and variations to keep the workout interesting and beneficial for weight reduction.

Seniors over 60 who understand and use these components in a chair yoga regimen can efficiently reduce weight while improving their overall health and well-being. Consistency and good form are essential for obtaining the intended outcomes safely and quickly.

Designing Routines for Weight Loss Goals

When establishing a weight reduction regimen, especially for seniors over 60, chair yoga is essential since it provides mild yet effective movements that are adapted to their needs. Start with a warm-up session that includes sitting stretches to relax muscles and stimulate blood flow. Next, use dynamic exercises like sitting twists and leg lifts to work core muscles and increase flexibility.

To target main muscle groups, transition to strength-building workouts using resistance bands or small weights. These may involve sitting bicep curls, shoulder presses, and leg extensions. As strength develops, gradually increase the number of repetitions and the resistance. To increase your heart rate and burn calories,combine aerobic exercises

Chair yoga positions, such as sitting mountain pose and seated forward bends, can be performed dynamically to add intensity. Encourage frequent activity to keep the heart rate up while remaining sitting.

Exercises that increase balance and stability can help you avoid falls and improve your mobility. Incorporate positions such as sat tree pose and seated warrior pose, holding them for many breaths to challenge stability and improve muscles.

Use relaxation and mindfulness practices to reduce stress and improve general well-being. Finish the regimen with sitting meditation or deep breathing techniques to relax the mind and body.

Maintain sufficient hydration throughout the program and promote a balanced diet rich in healthy foods to aid in weight loss. Monitor progress regularly and make adjustments to the program as needed to stay motivated and achieve results.

Designing a complete chair yoga regimen adapted to the individual needs of seniors over 60 will help them lose weight while also increasing overall health and energy.

Incorporating Dynamic Movements and Flow

To effectively include dynamic movements and flow into chair yoga for seniors over 60 who want to lose weight, you must engage the entire body while keeping fluidity in transitions.

Begin by focusing on movements that work key muscular groups such as the legs, arms, and core. To boost heart rate and promote circulation, perform sitting squats, leg lifts, and arm circles.

Encourage participants to transition easily from one activity to the next, stressing regulated breathing to improve calm and awareness. Maintaining appropriate form and alignment is critical for avoiding injury and increasing effectiveness.

Use props like resistance bands or tiny weights to increase resistance and intensity in the exercises, allowing seniors to gradually push their strength and endurance.

Incorporate dynamic stretches and mobility exercises to increase flexibility and range of motion, lowering the risk of stiffness and improving functional movement. Encourage participants to experiment with varied movement patterns and variations until they find what feels best for their bodies.

To improve proprioception and lessen the chance of falling, focus on balance and stability exercises like sitting spinal twists and side bends. Use smooth transitions between positions to enhance coordination and body awareness.

Tailor the intensity and complexity of the motions to the participants' particular requirements and skills, providing changes and alternatives as needed. Encourage elders to listen to their bodies and accept their limitations while still pushing themselves to grow.

By introducing dynamic movements and flow into chair yoga sessions for seniors over 60, you may offer them a pleasant and effective approach to increase their fitness, losing weight, and improve their general well-being.

Balancing Strength, Flexibility, and Cardiovascular Exercise

Balancing strength, flexibility, and aerobic exercise is critical for total health, particularly for seniors over 60 who want to lose weight with chair yoga. To begin, focus on strength training to preserve muscle mass and boost metabolism. Bodyweight exercises such as sitting leg lifts, arm curls with small weights, and chair squats will help you gain strength without strain.

Flexibility is also crucial since it increases the range of motion and lowers the chance of injury. Incorporate mild stretching motions into your chair yoga practice, concentrating on the neck, shoulders, back, hips, and legs. Practice motions like neck rolls, shoulder stretches, spine twists, and sitting forward folds to promote flexibility and mobility.

Cardiovascular activity is essential for burning calories and improving heart health. While chair yoga may not appear to be classic cardio, it may nonetheless raise your heart rate through dynamic movements and fluid sequences. Aim for constant activity, such as chair sun salutations or sitting marching, to get your blood flowing and burn calories.

To efficiently reduce weight, choose a balanced strategy that includes strength, flexibility, and cardiovascular training. Alternate between these components throughout the week for a well-rounded exercise routine. Pay close attention to your meals and hydration, since nutrition plays an important part in weight management.

Consistency is key commit to regular chair yoga sessions that include strength, flexibility, and cardio exercises. Listen to your body and alter the intensity as necessary, progressively increasing the difficulty over time. As a senior over 60, with effort and patience, you may reach your weight reduction objectives while also improving your general health and fitness.

Modifying Routines for Different Fitness Levels

When altering programs for different fitness levels, it is critical to personalize the workouts to each person's unique demands and talents. Several tweaks can assure safety and success for seniors over the age of 60 who want to lose weight with chair yoga.

First, emphasize mild motions that improve flexibility, balance, and strength. Begin with easy chair postures like sitting spinal twists and moderate side stretches to warm up the body and stimulate blood circulation.

Gradually incorporate more difficult positions as your strength and flexibility increase, but always consider safety above intensity. Encourage good breathing methods throughout the practice to increase relaxation and awareness.

To lose weight, integrate dynamic workouts that raise the heart rate, such as sitting marches or leg lifts. These activities can increase metabolism and burn calories without placing too much strain on joints.

Additionally, consider including resistance exercise with modest weights or resistance bands to build muscle mass, which can help increase metabolic rate and promote fat reduction.

Consistency is essential for any fitness plan. Encourage consistent practice, with at least three sessions per week, and highlight the significance of listening to one's body and accepting its limitations.

Provide adaptations and alternatives for positions that may be too difficult or uncomfortable, so that participants feel encouraged and empowered on their fitness path. Implementation of chair yoga routines to the requirements and abilities of seniors over 60, can help you in achieving your weight reduction objectives safely and successfully while also boosting general health and well-being.

Sample Chair Yoga Routines for Weight Loss

Begin chair yoga programs for weight reduction geared at seniors over 60 with easy warm-up movements. Sit tall in your chair, inhale deeply, and exhale fully, using your core muscles. Slowly rotate your neck from side to side, followed by shoulder rolls that softly raise and drop your shoulders.

Next, perform sitting twists to improve digestion and spinal mobility. Sit at the edge of your chair, feet flat on the ground. Inhale as you stretch your spine, then exhale as you slowly rotate to the right, with your left hand on the outside of your right knee and your right hand on the chair's back. Hold for a few breaths before repeating on the opposite side.

Continue doing sitting forward bends to stretch your hamstrings and lower back. Sit up straight, legs stretched in front of you. Inhale to stretch your spine, then exhale as you bend forward from your hips and reach for your toes or shins. Hold for a few breaths, feeling the stretch at the back of your legs.

Use sitting warrior postures to increase strength and stability. Sit tall, stretch your right leg to the side, and bend your left knee, placing your left foot firmly on the ground. Inhale while raising your arms aloft, extending towards the heavens. Exhale while leaning gently to the right, feeling the stretch on your left side. Hold for a few breaths before repeating on the opposite side.
.Relaxation and meditation should be the final steps of your chair yoga exercise.

Concentrate on your breathing after you close your eyes after seating comfortably

Inhale deeply, exhale thoroughly, and let your body relax entirely. Visualize yourself reaching your weight loss objectives while feeling powerful, bright, and healthy.

CHAPTERS SIX

Nutrition and Diet Tips for Seniors

Maintaining a balanced diet is essential for seniors' general health and weight management. Here are some thorough recommendations designed exclusively for seniors:

Prioritize nutrient-dense foods: Eat entire, unprocessed foods high in key nutrients such as fruits and vegetables, lean proteins, whole grains, and healthy fats. These foods include the essential vitamins, minerals, and antioxidants required for good health. Seniors frequently have diminished thirst feelings, so staying hydrated throughout the day is critical. Aim to drink plenty of water and eat hydrating meals like fruits and vegetables.

Mind portion sizes: As metabolism slows with age, it's critical to pay attention to portion sizes to avoid consuming too many calories. Use smaller dishes, bowls, and utensils to keep portion sizes under control and prevent overeating.

Opt for quality over quantity. Choose nutrient-dense foods over empty calories such as sugary snacks and processed meals. This guarantees that you obtain the greatest nutritious value from your food while eliminating extra sweets and bad fats.

Consider dietary constraints: If you have any dietary restrictions or medical problems, such as diabetes or high blood pressure, consult with a certified dietitian to create a tailored meal plan that satisfies your nutritional requirements while also managing your condition.

Now, let's speak about chair yoga, which is an excellent alternative for seniors over 60 who want to reduce weight and increase their flexibility.

Chair yoga consists of mild movements and stretches that may be done while sitting or utilizing a chair for support. It improves mobility, strength, and balance while also encouraging relaxation and lowering tension.

Include chair yoga into your daily practice by visiting courses made exclusively for seniors or following online lessons. Focus on activities that target different muscle areas, and strive for consistency in your practice to notice gains over time.

Ensure to listen to your body and adjust your exercises as needed to minimize strain or injury. Chair yoga, with dedication and patience, may be a beneficial supplement to

your weight reduction and general fitness
routine.

Importance of Nutrition for Weight Loss

Nutrition is essential for weight reduction, particularly for seniors over the age of 60 who practice Chair Yoga. To begin, remember that weight reduction is more than just decreasing calories; it is about providing your body with the proper nutrients while producing a calorie deficit. For seniors, this is especially important because metabolism typically slows with age.

A well-balanced diet rich in complete foods such as fruits, vegetables, lean meats, and whole grains provides vital nutrients for energy, muscle maintenance, and general health. These meals are also lower in calories, which helps you maintain your weight more successfully. They also include fiber, which promotes digestion and keeps you fuller for longer periods, lowering the possibility of binge eating.

Chair yoga is a mild kind of exercise that helps seniors improve their flexibility, strength, and balance. However, without sufficient nutrition, the advantages may be limited, particularly in terms of weight reduction. Nutrient-dense foods help your body recuperate from exercise, giving you enough energy to fully participate in Chair Yoga sessions.

Hydration is important for weight reduction and overall wellness. Drinking enough water throughout the day improves appetite regulation, digestion, and toxin disposal. Seniors sometimes have diminished thirst, thus it is essential to consume water regularly.

Avoiding processed and sugary meals is critical since they can contribute to weight gain and other health problems. Instead, look for entire, nutrient-dense foods. Portion control is also important, particularly for seniors who may have fewer appetites or have less active lifestyles.

Nutrition is essential for weight loss, particularly for seniors over 60 who practice Chair Yoga. You can successfully support your weight reduction journey and general well-being by feeding your body nutritious meals, staying hydrated, and being conscious of portion sizes.

Understanding Caloric Needs for Seniors

As a senior over 60 wanting to lose weight with chair yoga, it's critical to understand your calorie requirements. Your calorie demands depend on several aspects like age, gender, weight, height, exercise level, and metabolism.

As you age, your metabolism slows, which means you may need fewer calories to maintain your weight.Consider utilizing a senior-specific calorie calculator to assess your caloric needs. These calculators account for the metabolic changes that occur as you age.

Once you've estimated your daily caloric needs, you may change your consumption to generate a calorie deficit and lose weight.

Chair yoga might be a good workout for seniors who want to reduce weight. It provides low-impact exercises that increase flexibility, strength, and balance while being easy on the joints.

During chair yoga classes, you'll do a variety of postures and stretches that work different muscle areas. Although chair yoga may not burn as many calories as more strenuous types of exercise, it can still help with weight loss when paired with a healthy diet and frequent practice.

When implementing chair yoga into your weight loss routine, prioritize consistency and development. Aim to do chair yoga several times each week, progressively increasing the length and intensity of your sessions as your strength and flexibility improve.

Complement your chair yoga practice with aerobic and strength training to increase calorie burn and improve overall wellness.

Choosing Nutrient-Dense Foods

When choosing foods for good health, prioritize nutrient-dense selections. Aim for diversity by including colorful fruits and vegetables, lean meats, whole grains, and healthy fats in your meals. Choose minimally processed meals to increase nutritional intake and reduce empty calories.

Fruits and vegetables should be the cornerstone of your diet since they provide critical vitamins, minerals, and antioxidants. Include a variety of hues to guarantee a wide spectrum of nutrients.

Choose whole grains like quinoa, brown rice, and oats over refined grains like white bread and pasta to get more fiber and minerals.Lean proteins, such as chicken, fish, tofu, and lentils, are important for muscle repair and development.

Include them in your meals to improve general health and weight control. Don't forget about the beneficial fats in avocados, nuts, seeds, and olive oil, which are essential for brain function and hormone synthesis.

When practicing Chair Yoga for weight reduction as a senior over 60, concentrate on postures that raise your heart rate and develop muscular strength and flexibility.

Combining yoga postures with modest aerobic activities will help you burn calories and enhance your cardiovascular health. Use mindfulness practices to increase awareness of hunger and fullness cues.

Stay hydrated by drinking lots of water throughout the day, as dehydration is sometimes mistaken for hunger. Limit your intake of sugary drinks and alcohol in favor of water, herbal teas, and infused water for flavor without the extra calories.

Prioritize nutrient-dense foods for better overall health and weight management. When practicing Chair Yoga for Seniors Over 60, focus on moves that improve strength, flexibility, and cardiovascular health. To achieve the best outcomes, combine good eating habits with frequent exercise.

Healthy Eating Habits for Sustainable Weight Loss

To lose weight consistently, focus on healthy eating habits that are adapted to your specific needs. Start by focusing on nutrient-dense foods such as fruits, vegetables, lean meats, and whole grains. These foods include critical vitamins, minerals, and fiber, which help your body operate and keep you satiated.

To avoid overeating, keep your portion proportions under control. Mindful eating is paying attention to hunger and fullness signs rather than eating out of habit or emotion. Avoid missing meals, since this might result in increased hunger and overeating later in the day.

Maintain hydration by drinking lots of water throughout the day. Dehydration can be misinterpreted as hunger, resulting in excessive calorie consumption. Limit sugary drinks in favor of water, herbal teas, or infused water.

When it comes to chair yoga for seniors over 60, it might be a valuable complement to your weight reduction quest. Chair yoga uses moderate stretches and motions to increase flexibility, strength, and circulation. Additionally, it increases relaxation and decreases tension, which can help with weight reduction attempts.

Adding chair yoga into your regimen multiple times each week, aiming for at least 20-30 minutes each. Concentrate on activities that work specific muscular groups, such as the core, legs, and arms. Deep breathing exercises can help you relax and become more aware.

Check with your doctor before beginning any new workout routine, especially if you have any pre-existing health issues or concerns. With a commitment to appropriate eating habits and regular chair yoga practice, you may accomplish long-term weight loss and enhance your overall health.

Hydration and Its Role in Weight Management

Hydration is essential in weight management, especially when paired with chair yoga for seniors over 60. Water is needed for several body activities, including metabolism and digestion. When you are properly hydrated, your metabolism performs correctly, resulting in more efficient calorie burning.

Staying hydrated can help reduce overeating. Thirst can be mistaken for hunger, resulting in excessive calorie consumption. Drinking adequate water throughout the day might help you avoid misleading hunger signals and make better decisions about when and what to eat.

Water is essential for workout performance, including chair yoga. Proper hydration keeps your muscles and joints lubricated, which reduces the chance of damage during workouts. It also helps to keep your energy levels up, allowing you to exercise for extended periods.

Hydration is especially important for seniors who practice chair yoga to reduce weight. As we become older, our bodies may become less effective at maintaining fluid balance, making dehydration more likely. Dehydration can impair exercise performance and recuperation, reducing weight reduction progress.

Adding chair yoga into your routine is a wonderful approach for seniors to keep active and lose weight. Combining it with regular hydration has a synergistic effect that boosts. Hydration is essential for weight management, particularly for seniors who do chair yoga. Staying hydrated helps your metabolism, prevents snacking, and improves workout performance, all of which help you lose weight. So, keep your water bottle nearby and drink your way to a healthy you!

Practical Tips for Dining Out and Social Occasions

When dining out or attending social events, it is critical to keep your health objectives while also having fun. Here are some useful guidelines to assist you negotiate these situations:

Plan Ahead: Look up the menu online and select healthier selections. This way, you won't be tempted by less healthy options when you arrive.

Portion Control: Be cautious of your portion sizes. Opt for fewer servings or request a to-go box at the start of the meal to preserve half for later.

Mindful Eating: Take your time with each bite. Pay attention to your hunger cues and stop eating when you are full, not overloaded.

Hydration: Drink water during the meal to keep hydrated and regulate your hunger. Limit your intake of sugary beverages and alcohol, as they might add extra calories.

Balanced Plate: Aim for a meal that includes lean protein, veggies, complete grains, and healthy fats. Avoid fried or heavily sauced foods.

substitutes: Don't be afraid to ask for substitutes or changes to make your meal healthier. For example, replace fries with a side salad or request grilled instead of fried.

Share your health objectives with friends and family so that they can support your decisions and keep you on track.

Stay Active: Incorporate physical exercise into your daily routine, especially on days when you dine out. Walk before or after your meal to increase metabolism and assist digestion.

Chair Yoga for Seniors Over 60 to Lose Weight has several benefits. This low-impact exercise improves flexibility, strength, and balance, making it ideal for older persons. Chair Yoga can also help you lose weight by raising your calorie expenditure and encouraging you to be careful when eating.

Regular Chair Yoga sessions, combined with appropriate eating habits, can help you lose weight and feel better over time.

CHAPTER SEVEN

Motivation, Mindfulness, and Beyond

Motivation is the driving force behind every fitness journey, particularly for seniors taking up chair yoga. Set realistic goals that are meaningful to you, such as improving mobility, lowering discomfort, or increasing energy levels. Visualize yourself attaining these objectives to keep focused and motivated during your chair yoga practice.

Chair yoga for seniors relies heavily on mindfulness exercises. Practice mindfulness by remaining present in each movement and breath, letting go of distractions and judgments. Pay attention to how your body feels throughout each pose, noting any areas of tension or discomfort. Practice thankfulness for your body's skills and growth, which fosters a positive perspective and drives your enthusiasm to keep going.

Beyond drive and awareness, consistency is essential for success in chair yoga for weight reduction. Commit yourself to practice regularly, even if only for a few minutes every day. Consistent exercise not only improves your body but also maintains good behaviors that will help you lose weight.

Variety is essential for keeping your chair yoga practice interesting and successful. Investigate numerous positions and sequences to target specific muscle groups and push your body in novel ways. Incorporate moderate stretches, strengthening exercises, and relaxation techniques to improve general health and weight loss.

Listen to your body and respect its limits. Modify positions to accommodate any injuries or physical constraints. Remember that improvement takes time, so be patient with yourself and recognize tiny triumphs along the way.

Stay connected to a friendly group of elders who practice chair yoga. Share your experiences, struggles, and accomplishments with others who understand and support you. Having a support system might help you stay accountable and motivated to stick to your weight reduction goals.

Outside of chair yoga, practice good lifestyle practices such as nutritious food, water, and proper sleep. These elements complement your practice and help with general weight loss and well-being.

Chair yoga for seniors over 60 is a gentle yet effective approach to shedding weight and enhancing general health. Stay motivated, aware, and persistent in your practice, and you'll see physical and mental advantages.

*Cultivating Motivation for
Long-Term Success*

To build motivation for long-term success in chair yoga for seniors over 60 who want to reduce weight, it is critical to set clear and achievable goals. Begin by establishing your goals and breaking them down into smaller, more doable objectives. This allows you to monitor your progress and celebrate your accomplishments along the road, which keeps you motivated.

Discover activities inside chair yoga that you truly like. Whether it's moderate stretching, breathing exercises, or meditation, figuring out what makes you happy in your practice can help you stay dedicated in the long run.

Experiment with numerous positions and variations to keep your practice interesting and dynamic.

Another crucial part of keeping motivated is to surround oneself with a positive community. Joining a chair yoga class or connecting with like-minded people online may offer motivation, accountability, and a feeling of community. Sharing your experience with those who understand and empathize with your struggles may be extremely encouraging.

Rest when necessary, eat well, and make sleep a priority. Taking care of your entire health will not only benefit your chair yoga practice but will also increase your drive to persist with it in the long run.

It's also a good idea to remind yourself that chair yoga has benefits other than weight reduction. Consider how it increases flexibility, balance, posture, and general mobility. Celebrate the good improvements you see in your body and mind as you continue to practice.

Be patient and nice to yourself. Progress may be sluggish at times, but each stride forward represents success. Embrace the adventure, be consistent, and believe in your capacity to attain your goals through devotion and perseverance.

Practicing Mindfulness and Awareness

Mindfulness and awareness are essential for anybody, particularly seniors over 60 who want to reduce weight with chair yoga. Mindfulness entails being completely present in the moment and paying attention to sensations, thoughts, and emotions without judgment.

Awareness, on the other hand, requires perceiving these dimensions of experience and comprehending their implications for bodily and mental well-being. Mindfulness is essential in chair yoga because it helps seniors tune into their bodies and identify points of tension, discomfort, or constraint.

By being observant, individuals may alter postures to suit their requirements, avoiding strain and injury while still benefiting from the practice. Awareness contributes to a better knowledge of how various motions influence muscle activation, flexibility, and overall energy levels.

Encourage seniors to focus on their breath when doing chair yoga exercises, as it will help them pace their movements and deepen their connection with each pose. Mindful breathing not only relaxes the mind but also oxygenates the body, which aids in metabolism and weight reduction.

Additionally, attention and awareness go beyond the physical part of chair yoga. Seniors should be encouraged to monitor their thoughts and emotions throughout practice, identifying any self-limiting ideas or negative habits that may be impeding growth. Individuals who become aware of these mental habits might create a more positive mentality that will help them achieve their weight reduction objectives.

Consistency is essential when incorporating mindfulness and awareness into your chair yoga practice for weight reduction. Encourage elders to set aside time every day for practice, gradually increasing the duration and intensity as their confidence and abilities improve.

With patience and determination, they may use the power of mindfulness and awareness to not only lose weight but also enhance their overall quality of life.

Overcoming Challenges and Plateaus

Overcoming physical hurdles and plateaus, particularly through chair yoga for seniors over 60, requires creative techniques to maintain consistent growth and motivation.

First, recognize that plateaus are a normal part of any fitness quest. To overcome them, consider varying your routine. Incorporate a variety of chair yoga postures that target different muscle groups and motions to get complete exercise.

In addition, push yourself by progressively increasing the intensity or duration of your chair yoga practices. Consistency is essential. Set reasonable goals and stick to a consistent chair yoga practice regimen.

Even on days when motivation is low, turning up and participating in a brief session might help break through plateaus. Remember to listen to your body and alter the intensity as necessary to avoid damage.

Mindset is really important. Stay cheerful and resilient in the face of adversity. Instead of perceiving plateaus as setbacks, consider their chances for development and refinement. Celebrate minor wins along the road, such as learning a new position or noting increases in flexibility and strength.

Nutrition is another essential component. A healthy diet high in nutrient-dense foods can help your chair yoga practice. Stay hydrated and eat complete meals to provide your body with long-lasting energy for your workouts.

Also, seek help from peers or a certified fitness expert. Attending a chair yoga session for seniors may give accountability, friendship, and professional advice customized to your individual needs and restrictions.

Never underestimate the value of rest and recuperation. Adequate sleep and rest days help your body repair and renew, minimizing burnout and improving overall performance.

Implementing these tactics can help you overcome hurdles and plateaus in your chair yoga practice, ensuring that you continue to make progress toward your weight reduction objectives and general well-being. Stay dedicated, be patient, and remember that every step forward, no matter how tiny, puts you closer to your goal.

Celebrating Progress and
Achievements

Celebrating progress and accomplishments is critical for keeping motivation and momentum on your fitness path, particularly with chair yoga for seniors over 60 who want to reduce weight.

To begin, acknowledge every accomplishment, whether it's completing a set number of sessions or mastering a difficult posture. Recognizing your accomplishments promotes positive behavior and encourages further devotion.

Consider how far you've come since starting chair yoga. Consider improving your flexibility, strength, and overall well-being. Celebrating achievement fosters a sense of satisfaction and accomplishment, which boosts self-esteem and dedication to your fitness objectives.

Set attainable short-term goals to measure your development effectively. These goals might include extending the length of your chair yoga sessions or learning new positions. Celebrate each completed goal, no matter how minor, as it represents development and progress in your fitness quest.

Share your accomplishments with others, including friends, family, and your chair yoga instructor. Celebrating together creates a friendly environment and increases motivation. It also allows you to inspire and motivate others who may be on a similar journey.

Reward yourself after achieving key goals. Give yourself something special, like a soothing massage or a nutritious dinner at your favorite restaurant. Rewards provide positive reinforcement and help you stay motivated in your workout practice.

Always enjoy chair yoga's non-physical advantages, such as less stress, greater mood, and better sleep. These enhancements are just as significant as weight reduction and deserve appreciation.

Celebrating progress and accomplishments in chair yoga for seniors over 60 is critical for maintaining motivation and long-term dedication to your fitness objectives.

You may stay motivated and inspired on your fitness path by identifying milestones, creating objectives, celebrating victories, rewarding yourself, and recognizing non-physical rewards.

CONCLUSION

Chair yoga is a thorough and accessible way for seniors over the age of 60 to lose weight and improve their general well-being. Chair yoga, which combines mild yoga postures, mindful breathing techniques, and relaxation activities, provides a comprehensive approach to weight control in this group by addressing both physical and mental elements.

One of the key benefits of chair yoga is its versatility and inclusion. Seniors with varied mobility levels can safely engage in the exercise by using a chair as support, lowering the risk of injury and assuring a comfortable experience. This openness generates a sense of confidence and belonging in participants, removing entrance obstacles and fostering long-term commitment to the practice.

Chair yoga provides a doorway to physical activity for seniors who may have previously avoided traditional forms of exercise due to fear or difficulty. Chair yoga, which progressively introduces mild exercises and stretches, allows people to gain strength, flexibility, and balance at their speed, creating the groundwork for long-term weight loss and better physical function.

Beyond its physical advantages, chair yoga provides significant mental and emotional assistance to seniors in negotiating the problems of weight control. Mindfulness and meditation activities interwoven into each session can help individuals develop increased self-awareness, emotional resilience, and stress reduction. This mind-body link not only improves the effectiveness of weight reduction attempts but also promotes general mental health and a healthier relationship with food and body image.

The social aspect of chair yoga develops a feeling of community and camaraderie among seniors, offering important peer support and accountability throughout their weight reduction journey. Group sessions provide chances for interaction, shared experiences, and support, which strengthens motivation and commitment to reaching health objectives.

In essence, chair yoga is a holistic approach to weight loss for seniors over 60 that addresses physical, mental, and social aspects of well-being. Chair yoga encourages older individuals to regain agency over their health, build a deeper connection with themselves and others, and succeed in their quest for a better, more satisfying life by incorporating the concepts of accessibility, flexibility, and holistic wellness.

THANK YOU PAGE

Thank you for selecting this book. Your support is really appreciated. Similarly, I am grateful for the purchase of this book.

Your input is valuable; please share your ideas in a review. It serves as a reference for future improvements. Enjoy reading and utilizing it!

30 Weeks Workout Planner to Help Track Progress

	EXERCISE	GOAL
MON DAY		
TUES DAY		
WEDNES DAY		
THURS DAY		
FRI DAY		
SAT DAY		

Weekly Workout planner for seniors to lose weight

	EXERCISE	GOAL
MON DAY		
TUES DAY		
WEDNES DAY		
THURS DAY		
FRI DAY		
SAT DAY		

Weekly Workout planner for seniors to lose weight

	EXERCISE	GOAL
MON DAY		
TUES DAY		
WEDNES DAY		
THURS DAY		
FRI DAY		
SAT DAY		

Weekly Workout planner for seniors to lose weight

	EXERCISE	GOAL
MON DAY		
TUES DAY		
WEDNES DAY		
THURS DAY		
FRI DAY		
SAT DAY		

Weekly Workout planner for seniors to lose weight

	EXERCISE	GOAL
MON DAY		
TUES DAY		
WEDNES DAY		
THURS DAY		
FRI DAY		
SAT DAY		

Weekly Workout planner for seniors to lose weight

	EXERCISE	GOAL
MON DAY		
TUES DAY		
WEDNES DAY		
THURS DAY		
FRI DAY		
SAT DAY		

Weekly Workout planner for seniors to lose weight

	EXERCISE	GOAL
MON DAY		
TUES DAY		
WEDNES DAY		
THURS DAY		
FRI DAY		
SAT DAY		

Weekly Workout planner for seniors to lose weight

	EXERCISE	GOAL
MON DAY		
TUES DAY		
WEDNES DAY		
THURS DAY		
FRI DAY		
SAT DAY		

Weekly Workout planner for seniors to lose weight

	EXERCISE	GOAL
MON DAY		
TUES DAY		
WEDNES DAY		
THURS DAY		
FRI DAY		
SAT DAY		

	EXERCISE	GOAL
MON DAY		
TUES DAY		
WEDNES DAY		
THURS DAY		
FRI DAY		
SAT DAY		

Weekly Workout planner for seniors to lose weight

	EXERCISE	GOAL
MON DAY		
TUES DAY		
WEDNES DAY		
THURS DAY		
FRI DAY		
SAT DAY		

Weekly Workout planner for seniors to lose weight

	EXERCISE	GOAL
MON DAY		
TUES DAY		
WEDNES DAY		
THURS DAY		
FRI DAY		
SAT DAY		

Weekly Workout planner for seniors to lose weight

	EXERCISE	GOAL
MON DAY		
TUES DAY		
WEDNES DAY		
THURS DAY		
FRI DAY		
SAT DAY		

Weekly Workout planner for seniors to lose weight

	EXERCISE	GOAL
MON DAY		
TUES DAY		
WEDNES DAY		
THURS DAY		
FRI DAY		
SAT DAY		

Weekly Workout planner for seniors to lose weight

	EXERCISE	GOAL
MON DAY		
TUES DAY		
WEDNES DAY		
THURS DAY		
FRI DAY		
SAT DAY		

Weekly Workout planner for seniors to lose weight

	EXERCISE	GOAL
MON DAY		
TUES DAY		
WEDNES DAY		
THURS DAY		
FRI DAY		
SAT DAY		

Weekly Workout planner for seniors to lose weight

	EXERCISE	GOAL
MON DAY		
TUES DAY		
WEDNES DAY		
THURS DAY		
FRI DAY		
SAT DAY		

Weekly Workout planner for seniors to lose weight

	EXERCISE	GOAL
MON DAY		
TUES DAY		
WEDNES DAY		
THURS DAY		
FRI DAY		
SAT DAY		

Weekly Workout planner for seniors to lose weight

	EXERCISE	GOAL
MON DAY		
TUES DAY		
WEDNES DAY		
THURS DAY		
FRI DAY		
SAT DAY		

Weekly Workout planner for seniors to lose weight

	EXERCISE	GOAL
MON DAY		
TUES DAY		
WEDNES DAY		
THURS DAY		
FRI DAY		
SAT DAY		

Weekly Workout planner for seniors to lose weight

	EXERCISE	GOAL
MON DAY		
TUES DAY		
WEDNES DAY		
THURS DAY		
FRI DAY		
SAT DAY		

Weekly Workout planner for seniors to lose weight

	EXERCISE	GOAL
MON DAY		
TUES DAY		
WEDNES DAY		
THURS DAY		
FRI DAY		
SAT DAY		

Weekly Workout planner for seniors to lose weight

	EXERCISE	GOAL
MON DAY		
TUES DAY		
WEDNES DAY		
THURS DAY		
FRI DAY		
SAT DAY		

Weekly Workout planner for seniors to lose weight

	EXERCISE	GOAL
MON DAY		
TUES DAY		
WEDNES DAY		
THURS DAY		
FRI DAY		
SAT DAY		

Weekly Workout planner for seniors to lose weight

	EXERCISE	GOAL
MON DAY		
TUES DAY		
WEDNES DAY		
THURS DAY		
FRI DAY		
SAT DAY		

Weekly Workout planner for seniors to lose weight

	EXERCISE	GOAL
MON DAY		
TUES DAY		
WEDNES DAY		
THURS DAY		
FRI DAY		
SAT DAY		

	EXERCISE	GOAL
MON DAY		
TUES DAY		
WEDNES DAY		
THURS DAY		
FRI DAY		
SAT DAY		

Weekly Workout planner for seniors to lose weight

	EXERCISE	GOAL
MON DAY		
TUES DAY		
WEDNES DAY		
THURS DAY		
FRI DAY		
SAT DAY		

Weekly Workout planner for seniors to lose weight

	EXERCISE	GOAL
MON DAY		
TUES DAY		
WEDNES DAY		
THURS DAY		
FRI DAY		
SAT DAY		

Weekly Workout planner for seniors to lose weight

	EXERCISE	GOAL
MON DAY		
TUES DAY		
WEDNES DAY		
THURS DAY		
FRI DAY		
SAT DAY		

Weekly Workout planner for seniors to lose weight

	EXERCISE	GOAL
MON DAY		
TUES DAY		
WEDNES DAY		
THURS DAY		
FRI DAY		
SAT DAY		

www.ingramcontent.com/pod-product-compliance
Lightning Source LLC
Chambersburg PA
CBHW051603250726

48653CB00004BA/1312